"A Must Have Guide for a Healthy Lifestyle"

KEEP YOUR DOCTOR AWAY

BASIC GUIDE TO A HEALTHY LIFESTYLE

MALINI SENTHILMANI

First published in 2013

Published by DVG STAR Publishing

Copyright © 2013 Malini Senthilmani

ISBN-13:978-1494918675

ISBN-10:1494918676

CONTENTS

ACKNOWLEDGEMENTS

I would like to express my gratitude to the many people who gave me assistance through this book; to all those who provided support, offered feedback, and assisted in the editing, proofreading and design.

I would like to thank DVG STAR LTD in guiding me to publish this book. Without their guidance and support, I could not even think about publishing this book.

Last but not least, I would like to thank my son Mayooran & daughter-in-law Labosshy for guiding and encouraging me to write this book.

FOREWORD

Keep Your Doctor Away by Malini Senthilmani is a basic guide to a healthy lifestyle for the entire family. This book is a fantastic resource and user guide to help people to understand the nutritional needs that are essential for our everyday life.

This book enlightens the readers to how natural foods contain not only nutrients but also phytochemicals which are powerful antioxidants and how these help protect us from diseases such as cancer, diabetes, age related diseases like cataract and wrinkling of skin.

A lot of us are not aware of what sort of nutritional values are present within the fruits, vegetables and spices that we eat every day and which ones help prevent which disease.

Malini has also provided recipes of dishes in which these natural foods could be incorporated.

Reading though this book has helped me understand how important fruit, vegetables and spices are to a healthy lifestyle thus to prolong our life span. Having had over thirty years' experience in teaching biology and health sciences, Malini has broken down the information into easy to understand facts that were very interesting to read.

In this book:

You will learn the important facts about the different **nutrients, vitamins, minerals** and **phytonutrients** that are present in fruit, vegetables and spices.

You will learn the **health benefits** of various natural foods and how these help to prevent certain diseases earlier on in life.

You will also learn how to incorporate this into your daily routines, as Malini has provided very useful **recipes to guide you** in the right direction.

Labosshy Mayooran
MRes in Translational Medicine

FRUITS

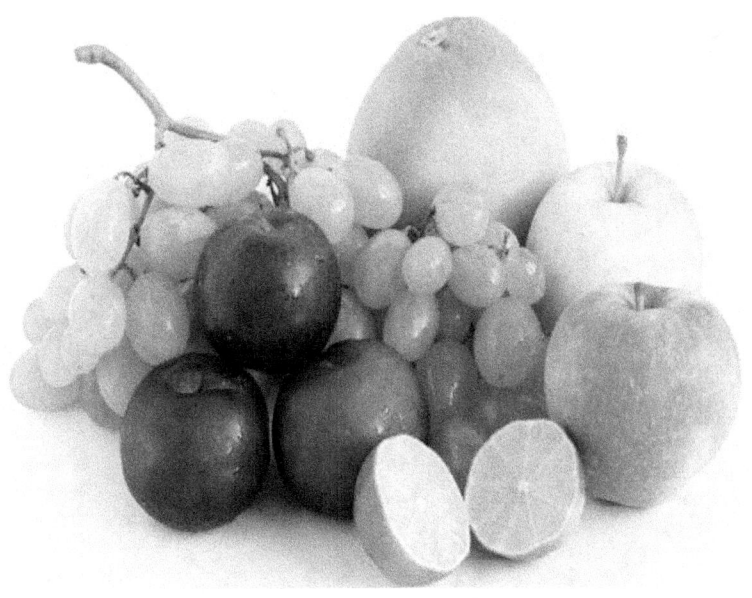

HEALTH BENEFITS OF FRUITS

Fruits are nature's wonderful gifts. These have a lot of vitamins and minerals, fibre and different phytochemicals. They are low in calories and fat. Think about these delicious colourful fruits: red, green, orange and yellow.

These differently coloured fruits have different phytochemicals which act as antioxidants that help to eliminate free radicals from the body. Free radicals are the main causative molecules that induce cancer causing cell proliferation. These free radicals form during metabolic activities in the cells due to environmental exposure to tobacco smoke, radiation, and some chemicals like mercury. These free radicals have the ability to damage the DNA in the cells and the protein in the cell membrane. This effect may cause the development of cancer cells in the damaged area.

Researchers have found that the phytochemicals in fruits, vegetables and spices act as antioxidants and detoxify these free radicals. Therefore if we eat these colourful fruits they will reduce the risk of diseases like cancer, heart disease, eye disease (cataract), and age related macular degeneration. They also reduce the effect of Alzheimer's disease, and delay aging and wrinkling of the skin.

The latest research has suggested that an element known as selenium is essential for the formation of an antioxidant enzyme that detoxifies free radicals.

Some fruits naturally contain selenium. Fruits act as natural vitamin tonics; if you eat at least one green, orange, yellow or red fruit and vegetables per day (that is, eat seven types a day) you can keep the doctor away and live a long, disease free life.

What are these colours? These colours are due to phytochemicals which act as powerful antioxidants in the human body.

Red fruits contain lycopene and anthocyanin, which are powerful antioxidant phytochemicals.

(These are in red grapes, red apples, and strawberries)

Orange and Yellow fruits contain lutein, zeaxanthin and carotenoids.

(In bananas, papaws, mangoes, oranges, lemons and, pineapples)

Green fruits contain phytochemicals like saponin and indole.

(In green grapes, avocados and green apples)

White vegetables contain allicin.

(In garlic and onion)

Purple/Blue fruits contain anthocyanin.

(In apples, grapes, and berries)

CHAPTER 1

APPLE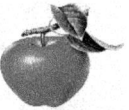

Nutrient	Value per 100g
Energy	50kcal
Carbohydrate	13.8g
Protein	0.26g
Fat	0.17g
Fibre	2.4g
Cholesterol	0

VITAMINS

Folate, Niacin, Vitamins B_5, B_6, Thiamine Riboflavin, Vitamin A, C, E and K.

MINERALS

Sodium (1 mg), Potassium (107 mg) Calcium, Iron, Magnesium, Manganese, Phosphorous, Zinc and Chromium.

[USDA national nutrient database, 2013]

BENEFITS

Apples are rich in vitamins, minerals and antioxidants, which are essential for a healthy life.

Apples contain soluble fibre called pectin which lowers high cholesterol levels in blood, helps in easy digestion and gives relief from constipation.

Acids in apples exert an antiseptic germ present in the mouth and prevent tooth decay.

Vitamin C in apples is a powerful antioxidant; it protects the brain from damage.

The antioxidant in apples is called quercetin; it reduces the effect of free radicals and protects the brain cells, thus reducing mental stress.

Apples can help prevent various diseases such as **cancer, heart disease, asthma, diabetes,** and **weight loss.**

Apples contain phytochemicals including quercetin, catechin, phloridzin, and chlorogenic acid, all of which are strong antioxidants. These phytochemicals may inhibit cancer cell proliferation, and regulate inflammatory and immune response.

Cardiovascular disease and cancer are thought to be

the results of oxidative stress. Apples are a good source of antioxidants. These antioxidants help to prevent oxidative stress and may therefore help prevent these chronic diseases. Apples contain quercetin, a powerful antioxidant which is associated with reducing the risk of lung cancer.

It was found that catechin, another flavonoid found in apples, is also associated with decreased epithelial lung cancer.

Flavonoids provide a 35% reduction in the risk of cardiovascular diseases and reduced risk of death from coronary heart disease.

Apple intake reduces the risk of asthma and decreases bronchial hyper sensitivity, therefore increasing lung function.

Higher quercetin levels may decrease the risk of type 2 diabetes, and the quercetin found in apples is considered to be associated with weight loss in overweight women.

APPLE SALAD

1 cup watermelon (chopped into half-inch cubes)

2 apples (chopped into cubes)

½ cup pineapple (chopped)

2 tablespoons raisin

Combine all fruits in a bowl and serve

CHAPTER 2

BANANA

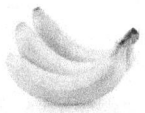

Nutrient	Value per 100g
Energy	90k.cal
Carbohydrate	22.84g
Protein	1.09g
Fat	0.33g
Cholesterol	0
Fibre	2.6g

VITAMINS

Folate, Niacin, Vitamins B_1, B_5, B_6, C, Riboflavin, Vitamin A, C, E and K.

MINERALS

Sodium (1 mg), Potassium (358 mg) Calcium, Copper, Iron, Magnesium, Manganese, Phosphorous, Selenium and Zinc.

PHYTONUTRIENTS

Alpha-carotene, Betacarotene and Lutein-zeaxanthin.

[USDA national nutrient database, 2013]

BENEFITS

Bananas are one of the cheapest fruits and are available throughout the year. This fruit is concentrated with easily digestible simple sugars that give instant energy. It is good for underweight children.

Bananas contain soluble fibre that helps digestion and provides relief from constipation. They have a high amount of potassium which is a component of body fluid and helps in maintaining heart rate and blood pressure by counteracting the bad effects of sodium. Bananas contain vitamin B_6 and Folate which are essential for the formation of red blood cells and help reduce anaemia. Vitamin K is essential for the clotting of blood. Calcium and phosphorous, on the other hand, help in strengthening bones and teeth.

Tryptophan is an amino acid found in bananas, which is converted to serotonin by our body. Serotonin helps in relaxing the mind, the brain, and the nervous system, and also regulates the mood, thus reducing tension of the body and mind, making one feel happy.

Thus phytochemicals such as lutein-zeaxanthin,

alpha-carotene act as antioxidants and reduce the bad effects of free radicals and protect the body. Carotene is essential for good vision and reduces the risk of night blindness.

BANANA MILKSHAKE

2 bananas chopped

1 cup of milk

1 tsp vanilla

1tsp curd

1tsp ground cashew nuts

Put all the ingredients except nuts in a blender and blend until smooth

Serve chilled, sprinkled with nuts

CHAPTER 3

GRAPES

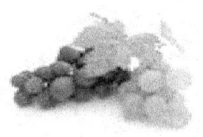

Nutrient	Value per 100g
Energy	69kcal
Carbohydrate	18g
Fibre	0.9g
Protein	0.72g
Cholesterol	0
Fat	0.16g

VITAMINS

Vitamin A, B_3, B_6, C, E, K, Biotin and Folate.

MINERALS

Potassium (191mg), Calcium, Copper, Iron, Magnesium, Manganese and Zinc.

PHYTONUTRIENTS

Alpha-carotene, Betacarotene and Lutein-zeaxanthin.

[USDA national nutrient database, 2013]

BENEFITS

Grapes have lots of vitamins, minerals and powerful antioxidant phytochemicals.

The fibre and organic acids in grapes reduce constipation and clean the digestive system.

Resveratrol, a phytochemical in grapes, increases the nitric oxide level in blood that prevents blood clots and causes relaxation in blood vessels, thus reducing the risk of heart attacks.

The iron content of the body is increased by regular consumption of grapes, which also reduces the anaemic condition of the body. The antioxidants in grapes help to boost the body's immune system.

Grapes help to eliminate uric acid in urine and reduce kidney stress.

Saponin present in the skin of green grapes prevents the absorption of cholesterol and reduces blood cholesterol levels.

Resveratrol is a powerful antioxidant that reduces breast cancer. It has been discovered in laboratory specimens that resveratrol reduces tumour cells. It also reduces prostate cancer by inhibiting the growth of tumour cells. Resveratrol helps to regenerate brain cells.

Grape juice helps to prevent age related macular degeneration in eyes and loss of vision.

Anthocyanin, a powerful antioxidant in grapes, has anti-allergic, anti-inflammatory, anti-microbial, and anti-cancer activity. Anthocyanin inhibits the growth of cancer cells.

It has been found that grape juice can cure migraines. It should be consumed early in the morning without mixing with water.

Grapes are very effective at eliminating toxins from the body and cleansing the blood.

FRUIT SALAD

1 piece papaya

1 apple

5 dates

Small piece of pineapple

10 grapes

1 teaspoon honey

1 teaspoon chopped cashew nuts

Chop all fruits and mix with honey

Serve chilled with ice cream on top

CHAPTER 4

PAPAYA

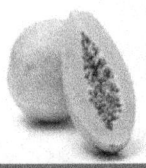

Nutrient	Value per 100g
Energy	39kcal
Fibre	1-8g
Carbohydrate	9.8g
Fat	0-14g
Protein	0-6g

VITAMINS

Vitamins B_2, B_3, B_5, B_6, C, E, K, Betacarotene, Biotin and Folate.

MINERALS

Sodium (3 mg,) Potassium (257 mg,) Calcium, Iron, Magnesium, Phosphorous and Zinc.

PHYTONUTRIENTS

Betacarotene, Crypto xanthene and Lutein-zeaxanthin.

[USDA national nutrient database, 2013]

BENEFITS

Papaya has vitamins A, B, C, E and K. They act as a tonic and rejuvenate the body.

Papaya has soluble fibre that helps easy bowel movement and reduces constipation. Papain enzyme in this fruit promotes the digestion of protein. In traditional medicine this ripe fruit was used to cure all kinds of stomach ailments and to reduce inflammation of the liver and spleen.

Potassium in this fruit is an important component of body fluid and helps in maintaining heart rate and blood pressure. Vitamin A in papaya is essential for healthy skin, mucous membranes, and vision.

Beta carotene and vitamin C are powerful antioxidants which help to reduce free radicals in the body and protect the body from the risk of cardiovascular diseases, as well as oral and lung cancer.

It has been found that vitamin A is essential for the visual cycle, reproduction, epithelial function, growth and development. Lutein is an antioxidant that protects the body from colon cancer, prostate cancer, and breast cancer. Betacarotene in papaw prevents the symptoms of aging and wrinkling of the skin and helps in maintaining glowing skin,

PAPAYA JUICE

Half a papaya, chopped

2 cups of water

1 cup of milk

1tsp honey

Put the ingredients in a blender

Blend well until smooth

Serve chilled

CHAPTER 5

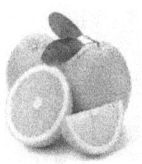

ORANGE

Nutrient	Value per 100g
Energy	47kcal
Carbohydrate	11.75g
Protein	0-94g
Fat	0-12g
Cholesterol	0
Fibre	2.4g

VITAMINS

Vitamin A, B_2, B_3, B_5, C, E, K, Thiamin and Folate.

MINERALS

Calcium, Iron, Magnesium, Manganese, Phosphorus, Potassium (169mg), Zinc and Copper.

PHYTONUTRIENTS

Alpha-carotene, Betacarotene and Lutein-zeaxanthin.

[USDA national nutrient database, 2013]

BENEFITS

Oranges are a citrus fruit, rich in vitamin C. Vitamin C is a powerful antioxidant that boosts the immune system of our body and induces disease resistance ability. High concentrations of vitamin C protect our body cells from the damage caused by free radicals. Orange juice induces the secretion of digestive juices in the colon, and helps in easy digestion and bowel movements, reducing constipation.

The pectin fibre in oranges is a laxative and protects the mucus membrane of the colon by decreasing the exposure to toxic metabolic products in the colon. The carbohydrates in oranges are fruit sugars that are easily digestible and give energy within half an hour. Orange juice, therefore, is a good kind of fruit juice for many types of fever. It has minerals which act as a tonic and cure fever.

Iron, folate, and vitamin B_6 are essential for the synthesis of haemoglobin and red blood cells in the blood. Haemoglobin is essential for carrying oxygen in the blood.

'Hesperidin' in the orange is a flavonoid type of phytochemical that reduces cholesterol levels in the blood and regulates blood pressure. High concentrations of vitamin C also maintain blood pressure.

Potassium in the orange is a component of body fluid. It helps in counteracting the sodium level in blood and maintains **blood pressure.**

Betacarotene a powerful antioxidant in oranges which protects the skin cells from getting damaged by free radicals, thus it prevents the symptoms of aging and wrinkling. It helps in maintaining **shiny skin.**

Liminoid, a phytochemical in oranges and the high concentration of vitamin C in oranges reduce the activity of free radicals and **prevent cancer in the mouth, colon, skin, lungs, and breast.**

Orange juice induces urinary output and reduces the risk of calcium oxalate stone formation in the kidneys; orange juice thus protects the kidneys.

Calcium and phosphorus in oranges keep bones and teeth healthy. Vitamin A is good for vision and reduces the risk of night blindness. Vitamin A, C, lutein, hesperidin and liminoid are powerful antioxidants that remove the free radicals' activity in the cells and protect our body.

HOW TO MAKE FRESH ORANGE JUICE

Peel 2 medium sized oranges

Cut into 4-8 slices

Remove the seeds

Put into a blender

Blend it for 30 seconds

Drain it to get pure orange juice

Add water to make one cup

CHAPTER 6

DATES

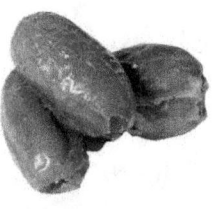

Nutrient	Value per 100g
Energy	273kcal
Carbohydrate	74.9g
Protein	1-8g
Fat	0.15g
Cholesterol	0
Fibre	6.7g

VITAMINS

Vitamin B_3, B_5, B_6, K, Betacarotene, Biotin and Folate.

MINERALS

Calcium, Copper, Iron, Magnesium, Manganese, Phosphorous, Potassium (696mg), Sodium (1mg) and Zinc.

PHYTONURTIENTS

Betacarotene and Lutein-zeaxanthin.

[USDA national nutrient database, 2013]

BENEFITS

Dates contain essential nutrients, vitamins, minerals, and antioxidants for healthy growth.

Dates are a good source of iron, which is essential for the synthesis of haemoglobin.

Haemoglobin in red blood cells carries oxygen all over the body. Dates are a good source of potassium, which is a component of body fluid that controls heart rate and blood pressure. The fibre in dates prevents low density cholesterol (LDL) absorption in the gut and prevents heart disease. It contains easily digestible sugars; when eaten they release energy and give strength immediately.

Vitamin A in dates is good for vision and essential for healthy mucous membranes and skin.

Calcium in dates is necessary for healthy bones and teeth, muscular function, and nerve conduction.

Tannin in dates has anti-infective and anti-inflammatory properties, and increases the immunity of the body. Betacarotene and lutein are antioxidants that protect the cells in the body from free radicals.

Zeaxanthin in dates is good for the retina and protects the eyes from age related macular degeneration. Lutein protects the body from colon cancer, prostate cancer, breast cancer and pancreatic cancer.

Dates have many vitamins and minerals and work as a tonic for all age groups.

DATE CAKE

INGREDIENTS

500 g chopped pitted dates
1 cup boiling water
250 g semolina (rulang)
1 teaspoon baking soda
2 teaspoon baking powder
1/4 teaspoon salt
250 g butter
200 g sugar
1 teaspoon vanilla, rose & almond essence
4 eggs
100 g cashew nuts, raisins, plums

PREPARATION

1. Stir together dates, boiling water and baking soda

2. Rest for 2 hours

3. Sieve flour three times with baking powder and salt to mix well

4. Cream the butter and roasted rulang together

5. Cream sugar and egg yolks together (in a separate mixing bowl)

6. Beat the egg whites to a foam (in a separate mixing bowl)

7. Mix all into the rulang & butter mix with a wooden spoon

8. Add chopped cashew nuts, raisins and plums and the cooled date-water mixture alternately to beaten mixture, till just combined.

9. Add all essences, mix well. Bake at 160°C for 45 minutes.

CHAPTER 7

POMEGRANATE

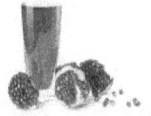

Nutrient	Value per 100g
Energy	83kcal
Carbohydrate	18.7g
Sugar	13.7g
Fibre	4.0g
Fat	1.2g
Cholesterol	0

VITAMINS

Vitamin B_1, B_2, B_3, B_5, B_6, C, E, K, Beta carotene, Biotin and Folate.

MINERALS

Sodium (3 mg), Potassium (236 mg), Calcium, Copper, Iron, Magnesium, Manganese, Phosphorous, Selenium and Zinc.

[USDA national nutrient database, 2013]

BENEFITS

This fruit is a good source of vitamin B complex, is a high source of other vitamins and minerals, and is considered a medicinal fruit. This fruit contains a large quantity of soluble and insoluble fibre, which helps in easy digestion and reduces constipation.

Pomegranates are a good source of vitamin C, a powerful antioxidant which helps the body develop resistance against infectious factors and inhibits viral infection.

Pomegranate juice contains ellagitannin, a tannin type of poly phenolic compound which is a powerful antioxidant. This removes free radicals from the cells and reduces heart disease risk factors. This juice reduces systolic blood pressure by inhibiting particular enzyme activity and reduces bad cholesterol levels in the blood.

Regular intake of pomegranate juice has been found to be effective against prostate cancer and diabetes, and ellagitannin can slow down the progression of cancer cells.

Pomegranate juice with honey is good for memory and the regeneration of brain cells. Anthocyanin, another phytochemical in this juice, is a powerful antioxidant, having an anti-bacterial effect and removes free radicals from the cells. The soluble fibre delays glucose absorption in the small intestine and helps to control diabetes.

POMERGRANATE JUICE

Grind the juicy seeds of one fruit

Add two cups of water

Add one teaspoon of honey to increase nutritious value

Serve chilled

VEGETABLES

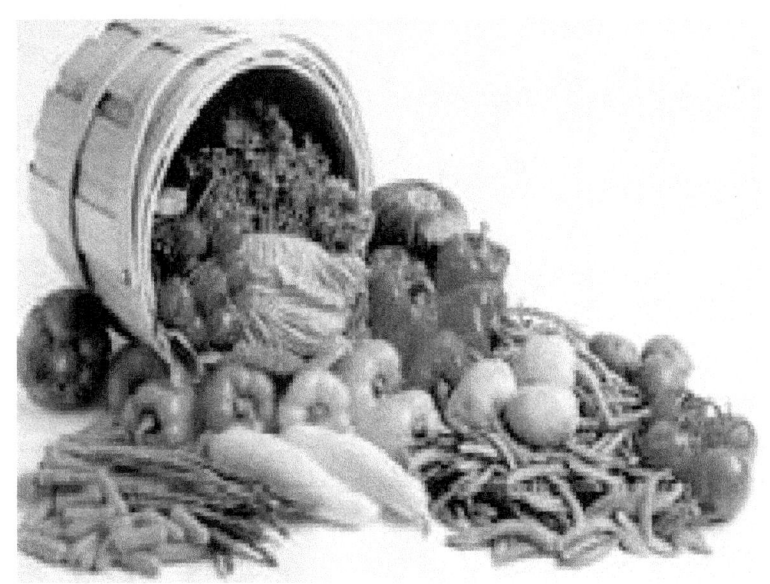

HEALTH BENEFITS OF VEGETABLES

Vegetables have a lot of vitamins, minerals, fibre, and phytochemicals. They are low in calories, fat and sugar. The differently coloured vegetables, green, orange, red and yellow, have different phytochemicals which act as antioxidants that help to eliminate free radicals from the body. These free radicals are the main causative molecules for inducing diseases like cancer, high blood pressure, diabetes, eye disease like cataract, and age related macular degeneration. Also phytochemicals delay aging and wrinkling of the skin. Micro elements in vegetables are needed to build new tissues, bones, muscles, blood cells, enzymes, hormones, and DNA. These elements are needed for all metabolic activities like nerve function, respiration, muscle contraction, enzyme activity and blood clotting.

Vegetables have a lot of soluble and insoluble fibre such as cellulose, mucilage, and pectin. These absorb excess water in the colon and retain moisture in the faecal matter, help in easy digestion, the easy movement of digested food, and help to reduce constipation, thus protecting the mucous membrane of the colon by decreasing the exposure time to toxic substances. Sufficient fibre in food gives protection from colon cancer and constipation. High fibre in foods helps to control diabetes, obesity and cholesterol levels of blood by decreasing its absorption in the colon. Recent scientific studies have shown that low calorie, nutrient rich foods help the human body to develop immunity and strength to fight against disease.

Most of the antioxidants in fruits, vegetables, and spices help to reduce cancer in the colon, lungs, breast, prostate and pancreas.

CHAPTER 8

BEETROOT

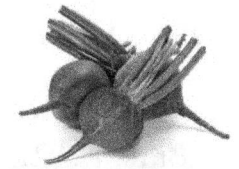

Nutrient	Value per 100g
Energy	43kcal
Protein	1.61g
Fibre	2.8g
Cholesterol	0
Carbohydrate	9.56g
Fat	0.17g

VITAMINS

Vitamin A, B3, B5, B6, Riboflavin, Thiamine, Vitamin C, K and Folate.

MINERALS

Calcium, Magnesium, Phosphorus, Potassium, Sodium, Zinc, Iron, Copper and Manganese.

PHYTONUTRIENTS

Carotene and Betanine.

[USDA national nutrient database, 2013]

BENEFITS

Recent research has shown that the high nitrate content in beetroot is absorbed by the intestine and is converted to nitric oxide in the body. This nitric oxide dilates blood vessels and reduces blood pressure. Nitric oxide helps in increasing blood supply to the brain and improves brain function.

Betanine in beetroot enhances the production of serotonin, a natural mood lifter in the body; beetroot can make you happy.

Iron and folate are essential for the formation of red blood cells and haemoglobin. This helps to reduce the anaemic condition of the body. Young beetroot leaves are a better source of iron. Recent discoveries found that folate is essential for pregnant mothers; folate is involved in the development of the spinal cord during first three months of pregnancy.

Vitamins and minerals in beetroot help in the production of new body cells and boosting the immune system.

Betacyanine in beetroot is an antioxidant which helps detox the liver, eliminates toxins and protects liver cells' DNA. Antioxidants help to remove free radicals and protect the cells from the risk of noncommunicable diseases.

Calcium is important for muscular and skeletal health.

Research has shown that drinking beetroot juice in the morning helps to reduce high blood pressure.

Lutein helps the health of the retina of eye, and reduces age related eye defects.

CHAPTER 9

CARROT

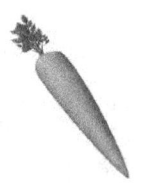

Nutrient	Value per 100g
Energy	41kcal
Protein	0.93mg
Fibre	2.8mg
Cholesterol	0
Carbohydrate	9.53mg

VITAMINS

Vitamin A, B3, B6, Riboflavin, Vitamin C, E, K and Folate.

MINERALS

Calcium, Iron, Magnesium, Phosphorus, Potassium, Sodium, Zinc and Selenium.

PHYTONUTRIENTS

Alpha-carotene (3427micro.g), Betacarotene (8285 micro.g) and Lutein-zeaxanthin (256micro.g).

[USDA national nutrient database, 2013]

BENEFITS

Carrots are rich in beta carotene, which is converted to vitamin A in the body. This vitamin A is necessary for good vision, reproduction, and the maintenance of epithelial integrity, growth and development. Vitamin A prevents cataracts and is good for skin disorders. Vitamin A and the antioxidants in carrots protect the skin from sun damage

Vitamin A prevents premature wrinkling, as well as dry uneven skin tone. It also flushes out the toxins from the body and reduces bile and fat in the liver.

Vitamin C helps the body to maintain healthy connective tissue, teeth and gums. It reduces the harmful effects of free radicals on the cells.

The high level of fibre in carrots helps in lowering blood sugar and cholesterol levels because the soluble fibres in carrots bind with bile acids and LDL. Fibre reduces constipation and facilitates easy bowl movements, which prevents cancer risk in the intestine.

High levels of betacarotene act as a powerful antioxidant that helps in protecting the body from free radical damage. Lutein helps in protecting the eyes from age related eye defects in elderly people.

The antioxidants in carrots fight against cancer by destroying cancerous cells in tumours.

There are high levels of minerals in carrots. Potassium is an important component of body fluids that helps maintain the heart rate and blood pressure by countering the effects of sodium.

Recent research has found that falcarinol in carrots acts as an antioxidant that reduces the risk of lung cancer, colon cancer, and breast cancer.

CHAPTER 10

TOMATO

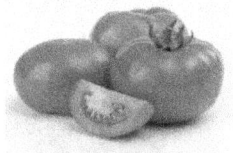

Nutrient	Value per 100g
Energy	18kcal
Protein	0.9g
Fibre	1.2g
Cholesterol	0
Carbohydrate	3.9g

VITAMINS

Vitamin A, B3, B5, B6, Vitamin C, E, K, Biotin and Folate.

MINERALS

Calcium, Iron, Magnesium, Manganese Phosphorus, Potassium, Sodium and Zinc.

PHYTONUTRIENTS

Carotene, Lycopene (2573micro.g) and Lutein-zeaxanthin.

[USDA national nutrient database, 2013]

BENEFITS

Tomato is a lycopene rich fruit. It has been found that lycopene reduces the risk of stomach, mouth, pharynx, colon, rectal, breast, and prostate cancers. Lycopene is a powerful antioxidant that acts against cancerous cell formation. Free radicals in the body can be reduced by lycopene which lowers the risk of heart disease, age related disease in eyes, and diabetes. Lycopene prevents skin damage from U.V rays and protects the skin. Vitamin C is a powerful antioxidant that boosts the immune system and protects the body from diseases.

Lutein and zeaxanthin protect the eyes from the age related macular defects in elderly people by filtering harmful UV rays.

Potassium in tomatoes helps control heart rate and blood pressure.

CHAPTER 11

CUCUMBER

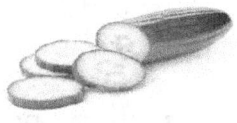

Nutrient	Value per 100g
Energy	15kcal
Protein	0.65g
Fibre	0.5g
Cholesterol	0
Carbohydrate	3.63g
Fat	0.11g

VITAMINS

Vitamin A, B_1, B_2, B_3, B_5, B_6, C, K, Folate and Biotin.

MINERALS

Calcium, Iron, Magnesium, Phosphorus, Potassium, Sodium, Zinc Manganese, Selenium, Fluoride, Silica and Copper.

PHYONUTRIENTS

Carotene and Lutein-zeaxanthin.

[USDA national nutrient database, 2013]

BENEFITS

The high water content of this vegetable promotes urination and prevents kidney stones, and provides cooling effect in the body. The good source of fibre in cucumbers helps in easy digestion. This vegetable can be used topically to relieve skin afflictions like sun burns and puffy eyes. Silica and antioxidants help to rejuvenate the skin.

Cucumbers are a good source of potassium which is a component of body fluid and maintains the sodium level in the blood, which reduces blood pressure.

Vitamin A and C, and betacarotene are antioxidants that reduce the effect of free radical damage in the body.

Cucumbers contain sterols which help to lower cholesterol levels in the blood.

CUCUMBER SALAD

Servings for 4-6 people

INGREDIENTS

2 cucumbers – thinly sliced
1 red onion – thinly sliced
1tablespoon lime juice
2 tablespoons plain yogurt
Salt and pepper to taste

PREPARATION

1. Whisk together yogurt, lemon juice, pepper
2. Mix in cucumber, onion, and other ingredients
3. Stir well and serve
4. Mix with yogurt mixture and chill till cold and serve

CHAPTER 12

OKRA

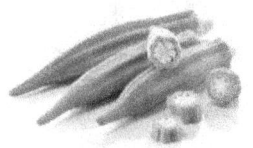

Nutrient	Value per 100g
Energy	30kcal
Carbohydrate	7.03g
Cholesterol	0
Protein	2.0g
Fat	0.1g
Fibre	3.2g

VITAMINS

Vitamin A, E, K, B_1, B_3, B_5, B_6, Folate, Riboflavin and Biotin.

MINERALS

Calcium, Iron, Magnesium, Phosphorus, Potassium, Sodium, Zinc Manganese and Selenium.

PHYTONURIENTS

Lutein and Carotene.

[USDA national nutrient database, 2013]

BENEFITS

Okra is rich in vitamins, minerals, fibre and antioxidants. The high fibre and mucilaginous content in okra helps in easy digestion; the soluble fibre in okra, called pectin, absorbs water and helps in peristalsis movement in the colon and relieves constipation.

The fibre in okra helps to reduce blood sugar by slowing down the sugar absorption in the blood.

Vitamin A is good for healthy mucus membranes and skin. Vitamin C helps the body develops immunity against infectious agents and reduces harmful free radicals. Folic acid in okra is good for nerve health.

CHAPTER 13

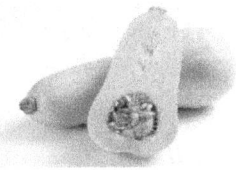

BUTTERNUT SQUASH

Nutrient	Value per 100g
Energy	45kcal
Carbohydrate	11.69g
Protein	1.09g
Fat	0.1g
Fibre	2 g
Cholesterol	0

VITAMINS

Vitamin A, C, E, K, Folate, B_2, B_3, B_5, B_6 and Thiamine.

MINERALS

Calcium, Iron, Magnesium, Phosphorus, Potassium, Sodium, Zinc, Manganese, Selenium and Copper.

PHYTONUTRIENTS

Alpha-carotene (4226micro.g) and xanthine (3471micro.g).

[USDA national nutrient database, 2013]

BENEFITS

Butternut squash is rich in dietary fibre, Vitamin A, folate, and antioxidants. Vitamin A is a powerful antioxidant that is good for maintaining the skin and mucous membranes. It is also essential for good vision. Vitamin A protects the body against lung cancer and oral cavity cancer.

Recent research has found that butternut squash has antioxidants that help in the prevention of prostate cancer colon cancer, and breast cancer.

Vitamin C helps to make collagen, which is a major component of cartilage which aids in joint support and flexibility. It is rich in carotene, lutein-zeaxanthin, and criptoxanthin, which are all powerful antioxidants that protect the body from free radicals. The seeds of this squash contain omega-6-fatty acids and oleic acid which are good for heart and brain health.

SPICES

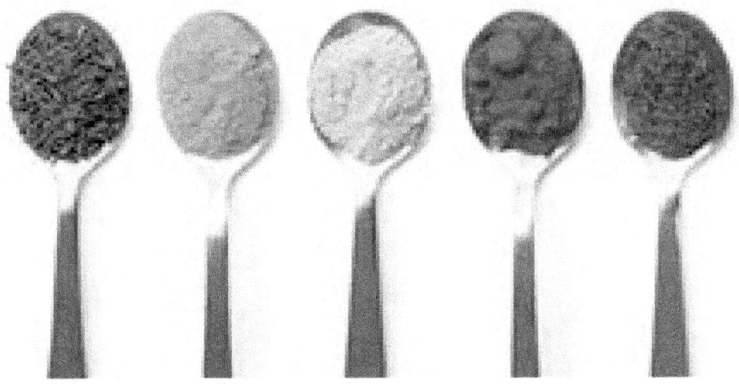

HEALTH BENEFITS OF SPICES

Spices are mostly used for taste but they have lot of minerals, vitamins, phytonutrients (antioxidants) and essential oils. Vitamins and minerals are essential for healthy growth and immunity of the body. Phytonutrients act as antioxidants which help to eliminate free radicals from the body. Free radicals are the main causative molecules for inducing diseases like cancer, high blood pressure, diabetes and cataracts. Garlic, onion and turmeric have antiviral, antibacterial, anti-inflammatory and anticancer properties.

CHAPTER 14

GARLIC

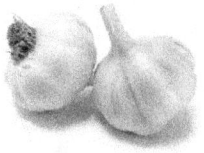

Nutrient	Value per 100g
Energy	149kcal
Fat	0.5g
Carbohydrate	33g
Protein	6g
Fibre	2.1g
Cholesterol	0

VITAMINS

Vitamin A, C, D, E, K, B_1, B_2, B_6, Niacin and Folate.

MINERALS

Calcium, Iron, Magnesium, Phosphorus, Potassium, Sodium, Zinc, Copper, Manganese and Selenium.

It also contains omega-3 fatty acid and omega-6 fatty acid.

[USDA national nutrient database, 2013]

BENEFITS

Garlic is an underground bulb vegetable used for flavouring in cooking. It contains many phytonutrients, minerals, vitamins and antioxidants.

Allicin, is a sulphur containing compound formed during enzymatic reaction in garlic when it is cut or crushed, and contains healing effects.

Studies showed that allicin reduces cholesterol production in the liver. Allicin releases nitric acid that relaxes the blood vessels' stiffness. It blocks the platelet clot formation in blood vessels and reduces coronary artery diseases.

Allicin is found to have antiviral and antifungal qualities; it reduces the formation of cancer causing substances. Clinical studies have shown that garlic reduces the risk of cancer in the stomach, colon, pancreas and breast. Antioxidants in garlic help destroy free radicals that damage cell membranes of DNA and decrease the effects of the aging process.

Selenium in garlic, a trace element, acts as an antioxidant and reduces free radical stress.

Omega-3 fatty acids are essential for brain functions such as memory and behavioural functions; it is essential for normal growth and development. Researchers have found that it reduces the risk of diseases like cancer and heart disease.

CHAPTER 15

ONION

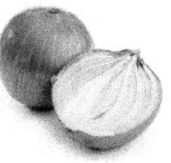

Nutrient	Value per 100g
Energy	40kcal
Carbohydrate	3.34g
Protein	1.1g
Fat	0.1g
Fibre	1.7g
Cholesterol	0

VITAMINS

Vitamin A, C, Folate, B_3, B_6, Thiamine and Riboflavin.

MINERALS

Calcium, Iron, Magnesium, Phosphorus, Potassium, Sodium, Zinc, Manganese and Copper.

PHYTONUTRIENTS

Carotene and Lutein-zeaxanthin.

[USDA national nutrient database, 2013]

BENEFITS

Onion is an underground bulb vegetable also used as a flavouring agent in cooking. It contains lot of vitamins, minerals, and antioxidants. Phytochemical allium is converted to allicin by enzyme activity. Allicin is an antioxidant which shows anti diabetic and anti-mutagenic property.

Laboratory studies have shown that allicin reduces cholesterol production in liver cells. Allicin has anti-viral and anti-fungal activity, which helps in boosting the immune system.

Allicin releases nitric oxide that relaxes blood vessels and reduces blood pressure, coronary artery diseases, and stroke.

Chromium, a trace element in onion, helps facilitate insulin action and controls sugar levels. Quercetin, a flavonoid in onion, is anti-inflammatory, anti-diabetic, and anti-carcinogenic activity.

Manganese and selenium are trace elements which are cofactors for antioxidant enzyme Superoxide Dismutase (SOD).

Iso thiocyanate in onion helps relieve colds and phlegm. Minerals in onions are essential for metabolic activities and healthy growth.

CHAPTER 16

PEPPER

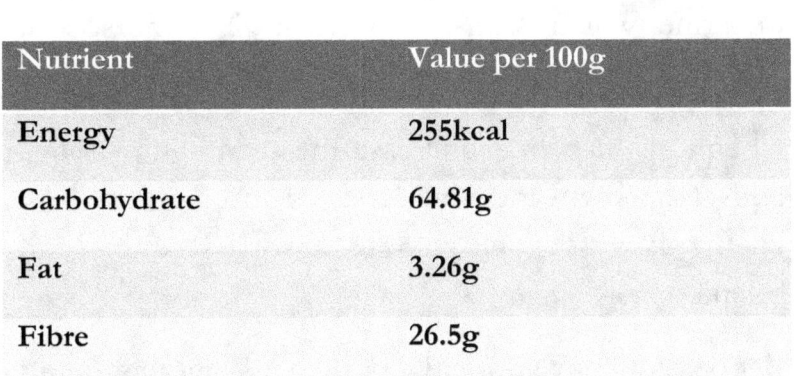

Nutrient	Value per 100g
Energy	255kcal
Carbohydrate	64.81g
Fat	3.26g
Fibre	26.5g
Protein	10.95g
Cholesterol	0

VITAMINS

Vitamin A, C, E, K, Folate, B_3, B_6, Thiamine and Riboflavin.

MINERALS

Calcium, Iron, Magnesium, Phosphorus, Potassium, Sodium, Zinc and Copper.

PHYTONUTRIENTS

Carotene, Lutein-zeaxanthin and Lycopene.

[USDA national nutrient database, 2013]

BENEFITS

Pepper is a dried fruit referred to as the 'king of spice.' Pepper contains an essential oil called peperine, which is an alkaloid that gives the special spicy character to pepper.

Chemicals in pepper increase the secretion of saliva and enzymes in intestine, and aid in digestion. The chemicals in pepper help to absorb vitamins and selenium.

Pepper contains antioxidants such as vitamins A and C, carotene, and lutein which protect the body from diseases and cancer.

Pepper contains a good source of minerals and vitamins that are essential for a healthy body and development.

CHAPTER 17

FENUGREEK

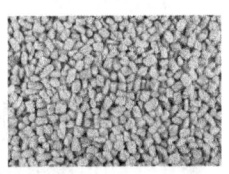

Nutrient	Value per 100g
Energy	323kcal
Carbohydrate	58.35g
Fat	6.4g
Fibre	24.6g
Protein	23g
Cholesterol	0

VITAMINS

Vitamin A, C, Folate, B_3, B_6, Thiamine and Riboflavin.

MINERALS

Calcium, Iron, Magnesium, Phosphorus, Potassium, Sodium, Zinc, Copper, Manganese and Selenium.

[USDA national nutrient database, 2013]

BENEFITS

Fenugreek is a dry seed used as spice in cooking, and contains a lot of mucilage which helps sooth gastro intestinal inflammation by coating the lining of stomach and intestine. This seed helps in cooling the body and reducing mucous in the sinuses.

Fenugreek contains soluble fibre pectin that facilitates bowel movements, relieves constipation and reduces colon cancer. It reduces blood cholesterol levels and protects the heart. The fibre in fenugreek helps in lowering the rate of glucose absorption in the intestine and controls blood sugar. These seeds can be used in a diabetic diet.

Phytochemicals in fenugreek, such as choline and yamogenin, show medicinal properties. An ammoniacal isoleucine acts on insulin secretion, and insulin controls blood sugar levels.

Vitamins and minerals found in fenugreek are essential for healthy growth and metabolic activity.

It is used in laxative, digestive, and inflammatory functions. It cures skin problems, sore throats and reduces menstrual pain. It has oestrogen-like properties and the intake of fenugreek helps to balance the mood.

CHAPTER 18

TURMERIC

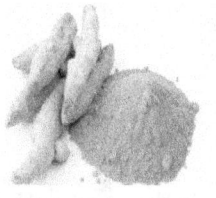

Nutrient	Value per 100g
Energy	354kcal
Carbohydrate	64.9g
Fat	9.88g
Fibre	21g
Protein	7.83g
Cholesterol	0

VITAMINS

Vitamin A, C, E, K, Folate, B_3, B_6, Thiamine and Riboflavin.

MINERALS

Calcium, Iron, Magnesium, Phosphorus, Potassium, Sodium, Zinc, Copper and Manganese.

[USDA national nutrient database, 2013]

BENEFITS

Turmeric is a yellow underground stem, and is used as a spice and disinfectant in Asian countries. It contains essential oils termerone and cucumin.

Cucumin is a polytphenolic compound which acts as a powerful anti-oxidant and also has antitumor, anti-ischemic, anti-inflammatory, anti-viral, and antibacterial properties. Small amounts of turmeric per day may help reduce anaemia and memory disorders and provide protection from cancer, high blood pressure, stroke and infectious diseases.

The American Cancer Society has suggested that cucumin in turmeric inhibits the growth of tumour cells in the colon, pancreas and prostate.

Turmeric contains a good source of vitamins, fibre, and minerals that are essential for healthy growth and development.

Turmeric is a good disinfectant and is used as germ killer in Asian countries.

CHAPTER 19

CHILI

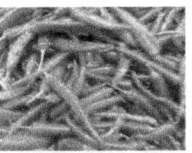

Nutrient	Value per 100g
Energy	318kcal
Carbohydrate	56.63g
Fat	17.27g
Fibre	27.2g
Protein	12.01g
Cholesterol	0

VITAMINS

Vitamin A, C, E, K, Folate, B_3, B_6, Thiamine and Riboflavin.

MINERALS

Calcium, Iron, Magnesium, Phosphorus, Potassium, Sodium, Zinc, Copper, Manganese and Selenium.

PHYONUTRIENTS

Betacarotene, Lutein-zeaxanthin and Cryptoxanthin.

[USDA national nutrient database, 2013]

BENEFITS

Chili is a fruit that is used fresh and dry in cooking. It contains capsaicin, an antioxidant that acts as an anti-bacterial and antidiuretic agent. It induces the secretion of saliva and digestive juices, and also induces taste buds in the tongue.

Chili reduces cholesterol levels in the blood. It contains vitamins A and C, as well as betacarotene and lutein which help protect the body from the effects of free radicals forming during stress and disease conditions.

TRADITIONAL SOUTH ASIAN HEALTHY DISHES

CHAPTER 20

ODIYAL KOOL

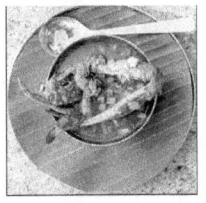

This is a tasty laxative that is good for clearing the intestine and encouraging bowel movements.

Odiyal is traditional soup in Jaffna Sri Lanka. This soup has become widely popular for a variety of spicy seafood.

To prepare odiyal flour: soak the flour in plain water for about 20 minutes and drain the water. Add fresh water and then drain the water. Repeat this 3 times to eliminate the bitter taste. Finally eliminate the water.

INGREDIENTS

½ cup odiyal flour, 15 long beans (cut), 15 jack fruit seeds (cut in half), 2 cups moringa leaves (or spinach leaves), small crabs – 4, medium prawns – 20, small fish – 4, 100 gm cuttlefish, ½ teaspoon turmeric powder, 2 tablespoons crushed dry chillies, 1 teaspoon tamarind paste, ½ cup cooked par-boiled rice, ½ teaspoon pepper powder, 4 L water, salt to taste

PREPARATION

1. Clean and wash the fish and cut them into pieces.

2. Clean and wash the crabs and cut into pieces.

3. Wash the cuttlefish and cut them into pieces.

4. Remove the shells of the prawns.

5. Wash and cut the vegetables.

6. In a large pot add water and bring to a boil.

7. Add the seafood, all the vegetables, and add salt to taste. Cook for 30 minutes.

8. Then add the chopped leaves.

9. Mix the prepared odiyal flour with the crushed chilies, tamarind paste and a little water.

10. Pour into the pot, and then add rice and salt to taste.

11. Keep stirring until all the flour is cooked and the mixture is thick and runny.

HOW TO MAKE RASAM

(This is good for colds and sore throats)

INGREDIENTS

2 tablespoons coriander

½ teaspoon pepper

½ teaspoon salt

1 teaspoon jeera (cumin seeds)

4 cloves garlic

1 red chilli

1 teaspoon tamarind paste

1 diced tomato

1 teaspoon fenugreek

PREPARATION

1. Take a pot and add 3 cups of water.

2. Add 1 teaspoon tamarind paste and salt to taste. Boil for two minutes.

3. Add 1 tsp fenugreek and 1 diced tomato. Mix well and boil for five minutes.

4. To the boiling mixture add finely ground coriander, garlic, cumin seeds, pepper, red chilli and boil for another two minutes.

You can drink this or eat it with rice.

REFERENCES

USDA national nutrient database, (2013). National Nutrient Database for Standard Reference, FOOD GROUP. [Online] Available from: http://ndb.nal.usda.gov/ndb/search/list. [Accessed 3rd November 2013]

BIBLIOGRAPHY

USDA national nutrient database, (2013). Dietary guidance for Americans, Balancing calories to manage weights. [Online] Available from: http://www.cnpp.usda.gov/Publications/DietaryGuidelines/2010/PolicyDoc/Chapter2.pdf. [Accessed 9th November 2013]

Jeanelle Boyer and Rui Hai Liu. (2004) Apple phytochemicals and their health benefits. Nutrition journal, 3 (5). [Online] Available from: http://www.nutritionj.com/content/3/1/5 [Accessed 28h October 2013]

Marta A Rieth, Marina B Moreira, et al. (2012) Fruits and vegetables intake and characteristics associated among adolescents from Southern Brazil. Nutrition journal, 11 (95). [Online] Available from: http://link.springer.com/article/10.1186%2F1475-2891-11-95#page-1 [Accessed 28h October 2013]

www.ingramcontent.com/pod-product-compliance
Lightning Source LLC
Chambersburg PA
CBHW060431290526
45791CB00002B/927